MW01296466

CPSIA information can be obtained
at www.ICGtesting.com
Printed in the USA
BVHW010221291018
531530BV00009B/194/P